FOOT REFLEXOLOGY COMPENDIUM

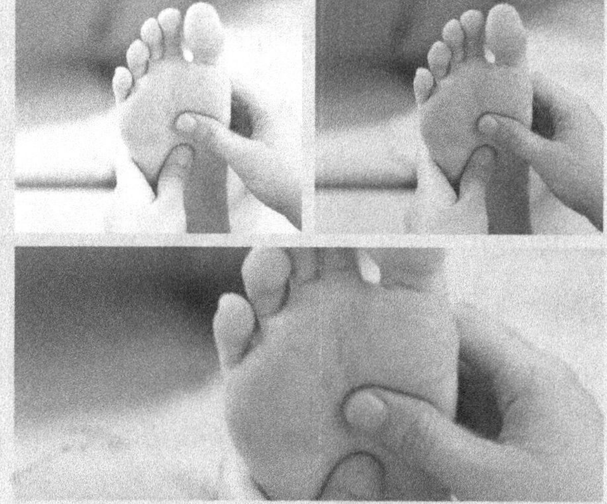

Dr. James K. Ferguson

COPYRIGHT © 2024 by Dr.

James K. Ferguson

TABLE OF CONTENTS

20 important things you should know about Foot Reflexology

Overview of Foot Reflexology

Brief History of Foot Reflexology

Benefits of Foot Reflexology

How Foot Reflexology Works

Understanding Reflexology

Principles of Reflexology

Zones and Reflex Areas on the Feet

The Connection Between Feet and Organs

Common Misconceptions About Reflexology

Getting Started with Foot Reflexology

Setting Up a Comfortable Environment for Foot Reflexology

INTRODUCTION

Welcome to the fascinating world of foot reflexology, where the ancient art of healing meets the modern science of wellness. In this introductory chapter, together we shall begin with the history, principles, and benefits of foot reflexology, setting the stage for your transformative journey into the realm of holistic health.

A Brief History of Foot Reflexology: The practice of foot reflexology dates back thousands of years, with roots in ancient Egypt, China, and India. These ancient civilizations believed that the feet were a mirror of the body, with specific points on the feet corresponding to various organs and systems. Over time, this knowledge evolved into the comprehensive system of foot reflexology that we know today.

Understanding the Principles of Foot Reflexology: At the core of foot reflexology are two key principles: the concept of reflex zones and the idea of energy flow. Reflex zones are areas on the feet that correspond to specific organs, glands, and body parts. By applying pressure to these reflex zones, practitioners believe they can stimulate the body's natural healing process and restore balance to the body's energy flow.

Benefits of Foot Reflexology: The benefits of foot reflexology are wide-ranging and profound. From stress relief and relaxation to improved circulation and pain relief, foot reflexology offers a holistic approach to health and wellness.

By working on the feet, reflexologists aim to not only address physical ailments but also promote emotional and mental well-being.

How Foot Reflexology Works: The exact mechanisms behind foot reflexology are still not fully understood, but many believe that it works by stimulating the nervous system and releasing endorphins, the body's natural painkillers. By applying pressure to specific points on the feet, reflexologists believe they can trigger a response in the corresponding organs or systems, promoting healing and balance throughout the body.

Your Journey Begins Here: As you embark on your journey through the pages of this book, you will learn how to harness the healing power of your feet and unlock a new level of health and wellness. Whether you are looking to relieve stress, improve your sleep, or enhance your overall well-being, foot reflexology offers a natural, safe, and effective way to achieve your health goals.

Join me as we explore the ancient practice of foot reflexology and discover how you can transform your health—one step at a time.

CHAPTER 1

20 important things you should know about Foot Reflexology

1. Foot reflexology is a holistic therapy that involves applying pressure to specific points on the feet to promote healing and relaxation in corresponding areas of the body.

2. Reflexology is based on the principle that there are reflex points on the feet that correspond to different organs, glands, and parts of the body.

3. Reflexologists believe that by stimulating these reflex points, they can help improve

circulation, reduce tension, and promote a sense of well-being.

4. Foot reflexology can be used to address a wide range of health issues, including stress, anxiety, digestive problems, and chronic pain.

5. Reflexology is a non-invasive therapy that is generally safe for most people, although it may not be suitable for those with certain foot conditions or medical issues.

6. A foot reflexology session typically lasts between 30 and 60 minutes and can be a relaxing and enjoyable experience.

7. Reflexology is often used as a complementary therapy alongside conventional medical treatment.

8. Regular foot reflexology sessions may help improve overall health and well-being by promoting relaxation and reducing stress.

9. Reflexology is suitable for people of all ages, from children to the elderly.

10. It is important to choose a qualified and experienced reflexologist when seeking foot reflexology treatment.

11. Reflexology is not a substitute for medical care, and it is important to consult with a healthcare professional for any serious health concerns.

12. Some people may experience discomfort during a reflexology session, but this is usually temporary and should subside quickly.

13. Reflexology can be a beneficial therapy for those looking to improve their overall health and well-being in a natural and holistic way.

14. The practice of foot reflexology has been used for thousands of years in various cultures around the world.

15. Reflexology is believed to help balance the body's energy and promote a sense of harmony and well-being.

16. Some research suggests that reflexology may be effective in reducing pain and improving quality of life for people with certain health conditions.

17. Foot reflexology can be a cost-effective and non-invasive way to improve your health and well-being.

18. Reflexology is a gentle and relaxing therapy that can be enjoyed by people of all fitness levels.

19. Many people find that foot reflexology helps them feel more grounded and balanced, both physically and emotionally.

20. Overall, foot reflexology is a safe and effective therapy that can help improve your health and well-being in a natural and holistic way.

CHAPTER 2

Overview of Foot Reflexology

Foot reflexology is a holistic healing technique that involves applying pressure to specific points on the feet to stimulate the body's natural healing process. It is based on the theory that these points, known as reflex zones, correspond to different organs and systems in the body. By applying pressure to these reflex zones, practitioners believe they can promote relaxation, improve circulation, and help the body restore balance.

The practice of foot reflexology dates back thousands of years, with origins in ancient Egypt, China, and India. These ancient cultures believed that the feet were a microcosm of the entire body, and by working on the feet, they could influence the health of the corresponding organs and systems.

In modern times, foot reflexology has gained popularity as a natural and non-invasive way to promote health and well-being. It is often used as a complementary therapy to conventional medical treatments for a variety of conditions, including stress, anxiety, chronic pain, and digestive issues.

During a foot reflexology session, a practitioner will use their hands to apply pressure to specific points on the feet, focusing on areas that correspond to the areas of the body where the client is experiencing issues. The pressure applied can range from gentle to firm, depending on the individual's preferences and needs.

Many people find foot reflexology to be a deeply relaxing and therapeutic experience. It can help relieve tension, improve circulation, and promote overall relaxation. Some people also believe that foot reflexology can help improve energy levels, enhance sleep quality, and boost the immune system.

Overall, foot reflexology is a gentle and effective way to support the body's natural healing process and promote overall health and well-being. Whether used as a standalone therapy or as part of a holistic health regimen, foot reflexology offers a natural and holistic approach to health and wellness.

Brief History of Foot Reflexology

The history of foot reflexology dates back thousands of years and is intertwined with the history of various ancient cultures. The practice of reflexology is believed to have originated in ancient Egypt, where illustrations on the tomb of Ankmahor, dating back to around 2330 BC, depict the practice of foot massage. The ancient Egyptians believed that applying pressure to specific points on the feet could alleviate pain and promote healing.

In ancient China, around 2700 BC, reflexology-like techniques were used as part of acupuncture and massage practices. The Chinese believed in the concept of "Qi," or life force energy, flowing through meridians in the body. Stimulating specific points on the feet was thought to help balance the flow of Qi and promote health.

Similarly, in India, the practice of Ayurveda includes a form of foot massage known as "Padabhyanga," which is believed to balance the doshas, or energies, in the body.

In the early 20th century, Dr. William Fitzgerald, an American ear, nose, and throat specialist, introduced the concept of zone therapy to the West. He divided the body into ten longitudinal zones and believed that applying pressure to specific points in these zones could relieve pain and promote healing in the corresponding areas of the body.

Eunice Ingham, a physiotherapist, further developed the concept of zone therapy in the

1930s and 1940s. She mapped out the reflex zones on the feet that corresponded to different organs and systems in the body, laying the foundation for modern foot reflexology as we know it today.

Since then, foot reflexology has gained popularity as a complementary therapy to promote health and well-being. It is now practiced worldwide and is often used in conjunction with other holistic health practices to support overall health and wellness.

Benefits of Foot Reflexology

Foot reflexology offers a range of potential benefits for both physical and mental well-being. While individual experiences may vary, many people report positive effects from regular foot reflexology sessions.

Here are some common benefits associated with foot reflexology:

1. Relaxation: One of the most well-known benefits of foot reflexology is its ability to promote relaxation. The gentle pressure applied to the feet can help relax the body and mind, reducing stress and tension.

2. Improved Circulation: Reflexology may help improve blood circulation in the body. By stimulating specific reflex points on the feet, reflexologists believe they can enhance blood flow to the organs and tissues, promoting better overall health.

3. Pain Relief: Foot reflexology is often used as a natural pain relief method. By targeting reflex points associated with pain, reflexologists aim to alleviate discomfort and promote healing.

4. Enhanced Energy Levels: Some people report feeling more energized after a reflexology session. The theory is that reflexology helps balance the body's energy flow, leading to increased vitality and well-being.

5. Better Sleep: Reflexology may help improve sleep quality by promoting relaxation and reducing stress. Many people find that they sleep more soundly after a reflexology session.

6. Stress Reduction: Reflexology is known for its stress-relieving effects. By relaxing the body and mind, reflexology can help reduce feelings of stress and anxiety.

7. Improved Digestion: Reflexologists believe that certain reflex points on the feet are connected to the digestive system. By stimulating these points, reflexology may help improve digestion and alleviate digestive issues.

8. Detoxification: Some proponents of reflexology believe that it can help the body detoxify by stimulating the lymphatic system and promoting the elimination of toxins.

9. Enhanced Well-Being: Overall, many people find that regular foot reflexology sessions contribute to their overall sense of well-being. It can be a relaxing and rejuvenating experience that helps them feel more balanced and centered.

It's important to note that while many people find foot reflexology beneficial, individual results may vary. It's always a good idea to consult with a healthcare professional before starting any new health regimen, including reflexology.

How Foot Reflexology Works

Foot reflexology is based on the principle that there are reflex points on the feet that correspond to specific organs and systems in the body. By applying pressure to these reflex points, reflexologists believe they can stimulate the body's natural healing process and promote overall well-being.

The theory behind how foot reflexology works is rooted in the concept of energy flow. According to traditional Chinese medicine, energy, or Qi, flows through the body along pathways called meridians. When this energy flow is disrupted or blocked, it can lead to illness or discomfort. By stimulating the reflex points on the feet, reflexologists aim to unblock these energy pathways and restore balance to the body's energy flow.

In addition to the energy flow theory, there is also the belief that foot reflexology works through the nervous system. The feet are rich in nerve endings, and by stimulating these nerve endings, reflexologists believe they can send signals to the brain and spinal cord, which in turn can affect the functioning of the corresponding organs and systems in the body.

Some studies have suggested that foot reflexology may have a positive impact on various aspects of health. For example, a 2015 study published in the Journal of Clinical Nursing found that foot reflexology was effective in reducing anxiety and improving quality of life in patients with multiple sclerosis.

Overall, while the exact mechanisms behind how foot reflexology works are not fully understood, many people find it to be a relaxing and therapeutic practice that can promote overall health and well-being.

CHAPTER 3

Understanding Reflexology

Reflexology is a natural healing practice based on the principle that there are reflex points on the feet (and hands) that correspond to every part, gland, and organ of the body. This ancient practice dates back thousands of years and is rooted in the belief that applying pressure to these reflex points can stimulate the body's natural healing process, promoting balance and overall well-being.

The concept of reflexology is based on the idea that the body is divided into ten longitudinal zones, each of which corresponds to different parts of the body. By stimulating these zones through the reflex points on the feet, reflexologists believe they can promote healing in the corresponding areas of the body.

Reflexology is often used as a complementary therapy to support overall health and well-being. It is believed to work by improving circulation, reducing stress, and promoting relaxation. Many people find reflexology to be a deeply relaxing and therapeutic experience, and it is often used to alleviate a variety of health issues, including pain, digestive problems, and stress-related conditions.

During a reflexology session, a practitioner will use their hands to apply pressure to specific points on the feet, focusing on areas that correspond to the client's specific health concerns. The pressure applied can range from gentle to firm, depending on the individual's preferences and needs.

Overall, reflexology is a gentle and non-invasive practice that can be used to support the body's natural healing process and promote overall health and well-being. Whether used as a standalone therapy or as part of a holistic health regimen, reflexology offers a natural and holistic approach to health and wellness.

Principles of Reflexology

Reflexology is based on several key principles that form the foundation of this holistic healing practice. Understanding these principles can help you appreciate how reflexology works and how it can benefit your health and well-being.

1. Reflex Zones: Reflexologists believe that the body is divided into ten longitudinal zones, five on each side of the body. These zones run from the head to the feet and hands and are believed to correspond to different parts of the body. By stimulating specific points within these zones, reflexologists aim to promote healing in the corresponding areas of the body.

2. Reflex Points: Within the reflex zones, there are specific points on the feet and hands that are believed to correspond to specific organs, glands, and body parts. For example, the tips of the toes are believed to correspond to the head, while the heel of the foot is believed to correspond to the lower back and intestines. By applying pressure to these reflex points, reflexologists aim to stimulate the body's natural healing process and restore balance.

3. Energy Flow: Reflexology is based on the concept of energy flow, similar to the principles of acupuncture and acupressure. It is believed that energy, or Qi, flows through the body along meridians or pathways. When this energy flow is blocked or disrupted, it can lead to illness or discomfort. By stimulating the reflex points, reflexologists aim to unblock these energy pathways and restore balance to the body's energy flow.

4. Holistic Approach: Reflexology takes a holistic approach to health and well-being, treating the whole person rather than just the symptoms of a particular ailment. By addressing imbalances in the body and promoting overall wellness, reflexology aims to support the body's natural healing process and enhance health on all levels - physical, mental, and emotional.

5. Self-Healing: Reflexology is based on the belief that the body has the ability to heal itself. By stimulating the reflex points, reflexologists aim to activate the body's self-healing mechanisms and promote health and well-being from within.

Overall, the principles of reflexology emphasize the interconnectedness of the body, mind, and spirit, and the importance of maintaining balance and harmony to achieve optimal health and wellness.

Zones and Reflex Areas on the Feet

Reflexology divides the body into ten longitudinal zones, five on each side of the body. These zones run from the head to the feet and hands, and each zone is believed to correspond to specific organs, glands, and body parts. Understanding these zones and reflex areas on the feet is key to practicing reflexology effectively.

1. Zone 1 (Head and Neck): The tips of the toes correspond to the head and neck. Stimulating these areas is believed to benefit the brain, sinuses, and upper respiratory system.

2. Zone 2 (Upper Body): The area from the base of the toes to the ball of the foot corresponds to the upper body, including the chest, heart, lungs, and shoulders.

3. Zone 3 (Digestive System): The middle of the foot corresponds to the digestive system, including the stomach, liver, pancreas, and intestines.

4. Zone 4 (Pelvis and Lower Back): The heel of the foot corresponds to the pelvis and lower back. Stimulating this area is believed to benefit the kidneys, bladder, and reproductive organs.

5. Zone 5 (Lower Body): The area from the middle of the foot to the heel corresponds to the lower body, including the hips, legs, and feet.

In addition to these zones, there are specific reflex areas on the feet that correspond to individual organs and systems in the body. These reflex areas are believed to be interconnected through the nervous system and energy pathways, and stimulating them is believed to promote healing and balance in the corresponding areas of the body.

Understanding the zones and reflex areas on the feet is essential for reflexologists, as they use this knowledge to tailor their treatments to each individual's needs. By applying pressure to specific points on the feet, reflexologists aim to stimulate the corresponding areas of the body and promote overall health and well-being.

The Connection Between Feet and Organs

Reflexology is based on the principle that there is a connection between specific points on the feet and hands and various organs, glands, and body parts. This theory suggests that by applying pressure to these reflex points, practitioners can stimulate the body's natural healing process and promote balance and well-being.

1. Nerve Pathways: The feet are rich in nerve endings, which are believed to be connected to the central nervous system. By stimulating these nerve endings through reflexology, practitioners aim to send signals to the brain and spinal cord, which can in turn affect the functioning of the corresponding organs and systems in the body.

2. Energy Flow: In traditional Chinese medicine, it is believed that energy, or Qi, flows through the body along pathways called meridians. These meridians are thought to connect the organs and systems of the body. By stimulating specific reflex points on the feet, reflexologists aim to balance the flow of Qi and promote health and well-being.

3. Microcosm of the Body: Reflexologists often refer to the feet as a "microcosm" of the body, meaning that they believe the entire body is reflected in the feet. According to this theory, each part of the foot corresponds to a specific organ or body part, and by working on these areas, reflexologists can influence the corresponding areas of the body.

4. Zone Therapy: Reflexology is also based on the concept of zone therapy, which divides the body into ten longitudinal zones. These zones run from the head to the feet and hands, and each zone is believed to correspond to specific organs and systems in the body. By stimulating the reflex points within these zones, reflexologists aim to promote healing in the corresponding areas of the body.

Overall, the connection between the feet and organs in reflexology is based on the idea that the body is interconnected, and that by working on the feet, practitioners can influence the health and functioning of the entire body. While the exact mechanisms behind how reflexology works are not fully understood, many people find it to be a relaxing and therapeutic practice that can support their overall health and well-being.

Common Misconceptions About Reflexology

Despite its popularity and widespread use, reflexology is sometimes misunderstood.

Here are some common misconceptions about reflexology:

1. Reflexology is just a foot massage: While reflexology does involve massaging the feet, it is more than just a simple massage. Reflexologists apply specific techniques and pressure to reflex points on the feet that are believed to correspond to specific organs and systems in the body. The goal is to stimulate these points to promote healing and balance in the body.

2. Reflexology is only for relaxation: While reflexology is known for its relaxing effects, it is also used to address a variety of health issues. Reflexologists believe that by working on the reflex points, they can help alleviate pain, improve circulation, and support overall health and well-being.

3. Reflexology is a cure-all: While reflexology can be beneficial for many people, it is not a cure-all. It is often used as a complementary therapy to support overall health and well-being, but it is not a substitute for medical treatment.

4. Reflexology is painful: Reflexology should not be painful. While some pressure is applied to the reflex points, it should not be uncomfortable. If you experience pain during a reflexology session, you should let your practitioner know so they can adjust their technique.

5. Reflexology is only for adults: Reflexology can be beneficial for people of all ages, including children and the elderly. It is often used to support overall health and well-being in people of all ages.

6. Reflexology is not based on science: While the exact mechanisms behind how reflexology works are not fully understood, there is evidence to suggest that it can have positive effects on health. Studies have shown that reflexology can help reduce pain, improve circulation, and promote relaxation.

Overall, while there may be misconceptions about reflexology, many people find it to be a beneficial and relaxing therapy that can support their overall health and well-being. It is always a good idea to speak with a qualified reflexologist or healthcare professional if you have any questions or concerns about reflexology.

CHAPTER 4

Getting Started with Foot Reflexology

If you're interested in trying foot reflexology for yourself, here are some steps to help you get started:

1. Learn the Basics: Before you begin practicing foot reflexology, it's important to learn the basics of the technique. You can find books, videos, and online resources that can help you understand the principles and techniques of reflexology.

2. Find a Qualified Reflexologist: If you're new to reflexology, it may be helpful to schedule a session with a qualified reflexologist. This can give you a better understanding of how reflexology works and what to expect during a session.

3. Gather Your Supplies: To practice foot reflexology at home, you'll need a few supplies, including a comfortable chair, a foot bath or basin, a towel, and some lotion or oil for massage.

4. Prepare Your Space: Find a quiet and comfortable place where you can relax and focus on your feet. Set up your chair and foot bath, and gather your supplies.

5. Begin with a Foot Soak: Start by soaking your feet in warm water for 10-15 minutes. This can help relax your muscles and prepare your feet for the reflexology treatment.

6. Apply Lotion or Oil: After soaking, dry your feet and apply a small amount of lotion or oil to your hands. Gently massage your feet, paying attention to any areas of tension or discomfort.

7. Identify Reflex Points: Use a reflexology chart to identify the reflex points on your feet that correspond to different organs and systems in the body.

8. Apply Pressure: Using your thumbs or fingers, apply gentle pressure to the reflex points on your feet. Use a firm but gentle pressure, and avoid pressing too hard or causing discomfort.

9. Work the Entire Foot: Work your way around the entire foot, paying attention to each reflex point. Spend extra time on areas that feel tender or tense.

10. Relax and Enjoy: Reflexology is a relaxing and therapeutic practice. Take your time and enjoy the experience. After you finish, take a few moments to relax and allow the effects of the reflexology treatment to sink in.

By following these steps, you can begin to experience the benefits of foot reflexology and incorporate this ancient practice into your wellness routine.

Setting Up a Comfortable Environment for Foot Reflexology

Creating a comfortable environment is essential for a relaxing and effective foot reflexology session.

Here are some tips to help you set up a comfortable space:

1. Choose a Quiet Space: Find a quiet and peaceful area where you can relax without distractions. This could be a bedroom, living room, or any other space where you feel comfortable.

2. Use Comfortable Furniture: Use a comfortable chair or recliner where you can sit comfortably with your feet up. Make sure the chair provides adequate support for your back and arms.

3. Gather Supplies: Gather all the supplies you'll need for your reflexology session, including a foot bath or basin, towels, lotion or oil, and any other tools or accessories you plan to use.

4. Set the Mood: Create a relaxing atmosphere with soft lighting, calming music, and pleasant scents. You may also want to use candles or essential oils to enhance the ambiance.

5. Prepare Your Feet: Before beginning your reflexology session, soak your feet in warm water for 10-15 minutes. This can help relax your muscles and prepare your feet for the treatment.

6. Use Supportive Pillows: If needed, use pillows or cushions to support your back, neck, and feet during the session. This can help you maintain a comfortable position throughout the treatment.

7. Eliminate Distractions: Turn off your phone and any other devices that could interrupt your session. Create a peaceful environment where you can fully relax and focus on the reflexology treatment.

8. Maintain a Comfortable Temperature: Make sure the room is at a comfortable temperature, neither too hot nor too cold. This will help you relax and enjoy the treatment.

9. Stay Hydrated: Have a glass of water nearby to stay hydrated during your session. Drinking water can help flush out toxins and promote overall well-being.

10. Practice Mindfulness: As you perform the reflexology treatment, stay present and mindful of the sensations in your feet. Focus on your breathing and allow yourself to fully relax and enjoy the experience.

By creating a comfortable environment for your foot reflexology session, you can enhance the effectiveness of the treatment and promote a deeper sense of relaxation and well-being.

Tools and Equipment Needed for Foot Reflexology

To perform foot reflexology effectively, you'll need a few basic tools and equipment.

Here's a list of what you'll need:

1. Reflexology Chart: A reflexology chart is a visual guide that shows the reflex points on the feet and their corresponding organs and body parts. This chart is essential for identifying the reflex points during a reflexology session.

2. Chair or Recliner: You'll need a comfortable chair or recliner where the person receiving the reflexology treatment can sit comfortably with their feet up. The chair should provide adequate support for the back and arms.

3. Foot Bath or Basin: A foot bath or basin filled with warm water can help relax the feet before the reflexology treatment. Adding Epsom salts or essential oils to the water can enhance the relaxation benefits.

4. Towels: Have a few towels on hand to dry the feet after soaking and to clean up any excess lotion or oil during the treatment.

5. Lotion or Oil: Use a small amount of lotion or oil to massage the feet during the reflexology treatment. This can help reduce friction and enhance the relaxation benefits.

6. Timer: A timer can be helpful for keeping track of the duration of the reflexology treatment. Most sessions last between 30 to 60 minutes, depending on the individual's needs.

7. Reflexology Tools: While not necessary, some reflexologists use specialized tools to apply pressure to the reflex points on the feet. These tools can include wooden or rubber tools designed specifically for reflexology.

8. Comfortable Pillows: Use pillows or cushions to support the back, neck, and feet of the person receiving the reflexology treatment. This can help them maintain a comfortable position throughout the session.

9. Music Player: Playing calming music during the reflexology session can enhance the relaxation benefits and create a peaceful atmosphere.

10. Optional: Essential Oils or Aromatherapy Diffuser: Using essential oils or an aromatherapy diffuser can enhance the relaxation benefits of the reflexology treatment. Choose oils with calming and soothing properties, such as lavender or chamomile.

By having these tools and equipment on hand, you can create a comfortable and relaxing environment for performing foot reflexology and enhance the overall effectiveness of the treatment.

Safety Precautions and Contraindications for Foot Reflexology

While foot reflexology is generally safe for most people, there are some precautions and contraindications to keep in mind to ensure a safe and effective treatment.

Here are some safety precautions and contraindications for foot reflexology:

1. Pregnancy: Reflexology is generally safe during pregnancy, but it's important to avoid certain reflex points that are believed to stimulate uterine contractions. Pregnant women should seek guidance from a qualified reflexologist who is experienced in treating pregnant women.

2. Medical Conditions: People with certain medical conditions, such as diabetes, epilepsy, or heart problems, should consult with their healthcare provider before receiving reflexology. Reflexology may affect blood sugar levels, trigger seizures, or affect heart function in some individuals.

3. Foot Injuries or Infections: People with foot injuries, infections, or open wounds should avoid reflexology until the condition has healed. Reflexology may exacerbate these conditions or introduce bacteria into open wounds.

4. Blood Clotting Disorders: People with blood clotting disorders should avoid reflexology, as the pressure applied to the feet during treatment could potentially cause bruising or other complications.

5. Recent Surgeries: People who have recently undergone surgery should wait until they have fully recovered before receiving reflexology. Reflexology may interfere with the healing process or cause discomfort in the surgical area.

6. Allergies: People with allergies to lotions, oils, or other products used during reflexology should inform their reflexologist before the treatment begins.

7. Discomfort or Pain: Reflexology should not be painful. If you experience any discomfort or pain during the treatment, inform your reflexologist immediately. They can adjust their technique to ensure your comfort.

8. Hygiene: Ensure that the reflexologist washes their hands before beginning the treatment and that all equipment and tools used are clean and sanitized.

9. Communication: Communicate openly with your reflexologist about any health concerns or conditions you have. This will help them tailor the treatment to meet your individual needs and ensure your safety.

By following these safety precautions and contraindications, you can enjoy the benefits of foot reflexology in a safe and effective manner. Always consult with a qualified reflexologist or healthcare provider if you have any concerns about receiving reflexology.

CHAPTER 5

Techniques of Foot Reflexology

Foot reflexology involves applying pressure to specific points on the feet to stimulate the body's natural healing process.

There are several techniques used in foot reflexology to achieve this, including:

1. Thumb Walking: This technique involves using the thumbs to apply steady pressure to the reflex points on the feet. The reflexologist uses a walking motion, moving from the heel to the toes and back again, to stimulate the reflex points.

2. Finger Walking: Similar to thumb walking, finger walking involves using the fingers to apply pressure to the reflex points on the feet. This technique is often used to target specific points that may be more easily accessed with the fingers than with the thumbs.

3. Rotational Pressing: In this technique, the reflexologist uses the thumbs or fingers to apply a rotating motion to the reflex points. This can help release tension and stimulate the flow of energy in the body.

4. Hooking In: This technique involves using the fingers to hook into a specific reflex point and apply pressure. This can be useful for targeting specific points that may be tender or in need of extra attention.

5. Finger and Thumb Walking: Combining thumb walking and finger walking, this technique involves using both the thumbs and fingers to apply pressure to the reflex points. This can provide a more thorough and effective treatment.

6. Kneading: Similar to kneading dough, this technique involves using the thumbs or fingers to gently knead the reflex points on the feet. This can help release tension and promote relaxation.

7. Rotating Joints: This technique involves gently rotating the joints of the toes and ankles to help improve mobility and flexibility. This can be particularly beneficial for people with stiff or sore joints.

8. Flexing and Extending: This technique involves flexing and extending the toes and ankles to help improve circulation and stimulate the reflex points. This can help relieve tension and promote relaxation in the feet.

9. Circular Frictions: This technique involves using the thumbs or fingers to apply small circular motions to the reflex points. This can help stimulate the reflex points and promote healing in the corresponding areas of the body.

These are just a few of the techniques used in foot reflexology. A qualified reflexologist will tailor the treatment to meet your individual needs, using a combination of techniques to achieve the best results.

Basic Foot Reflexology Techniques

Foot reflexology involves applying pressure to specific points on the feet to stimulate the body's natural healing process.

Here are some basic techniques used in foot reflexology:

1. Thumb Walking: Use your thumbs to apply gentle pressure to the reflex points on the feet. Start at the base of the big toe and move in a walking motion towards the heel. Repeat this motion for each toe and the areas between the toes.

2. Finger Walking: Similar to thumb walking, use your fingers to apply pressure to the reflex points on the feet. This technique can be useful for targeting smaller areas or areas that are difficult to reach with your thumbs.

3. Rotational Pressing: Use your thumbs or fingers to apply a rotating motion to the reflex points. This can help release tension and stimulate the flow of energy in the body.

4. Hooking In: Use your fingers to hook into a specific reflex point and apply pressure. This technique can be useful for targeting specific points that may be tender or in need of extra attention.

5. Kneading: Gently knead the reflex points on the feet using your thumbs or fingers. This can help release tension and promote relaxation.

6. Flexing and Extending: Flex and extend the toes and ankles to help improve circulation and stimulate the reflex points. This can help relieve tension and promote relaxation in the feet.

7. Circular Frictions: Use your thumbs or fingers to apply small circular motions to the reflex points. This can help stimulate the reflex points and promote healing in the corresponding areas of the body.

These basic techniques can be used alone or in combination to provide a relaxing and therapeutic foot reflexology treatment. Adjust the pressure and speed of your movements to suit the comfort level of the person receiving the treatment.

Advanced Foot Reflexology Techniques

Advanced foot reflexology techniques build upon the basic techniques and involve more specific and targeted approaches to address various health issues.

Here are some advanced techniques used in foot reflexology:

1. Cross-Thumb Technique: This technique involves using the thumbs to apply pressure to opposite sides of a reflex point simultaneously. This can help stimulate the reflex point more effectively and provide deeper relief.

2. Finger Rotation Technique: Use your fingers to gently rotate the skin around a reflex point in a circular motion. This can help release tension and improve circulation in the area.

3. Zone Tapping: This technique involves using your fingertips to tap lightly along the longitudinal zones of the foot. This can help stimulate the nerve endings and promote energy flow along the meridians.

4. Knuckle Rotation Technique: Use your knuckles to apply gentle pressure to a reflex point and then rotate them in a circular motion. This can help release tension and stimulate the reflex point more deeply.

5. Thumb and Finger Walking Combination: Combine thumb walking and finger walking to target multiple reflex points simultaneously.

This can help provide a more comprehensive treatment and address a wider range of issues.

6. Toe Rotation Technique: Gently rotate each toe in a circular motion to help release tension and stimulate the reflex points in the toes.

7. Heel Slide Technique: Use your thumbs to apply pressure to the heel of the foot and then slide them towards the toes. This can help stimulate the reflex points along the bottom of the foot.

8. Reflex Point Compression: Apply firm pressure to a specific reflex point for a few seconds and then release. Repeat this process several times to help stimulate the reflex point and promote healing.

These advanced techniques should be used with caution and only by experienced reflexologists. It's important to tailor the treatment to the individual's needs and comfort level to ensure a safe and effective session.

Incorporating Essential Oils and Aromatherapy in Foot Reflexology

Essential oils and aromatherapy can enhance the benefits of foot reflexology by promoting relaxation, reducing stress, and supporting overall well-being.

Here's how you can incorporate essential oils and aromatherapy into your foot reflexology practice:

1. Choose the Right Essential Oils: Select essential oils that are known for their relaxing and therapeutic properties. Lavender, chamomile, peppermint, and eucalyptus are popular choices for foot reflexology.

2. Dilute the Essential Oils: Essential oils are highly concentrated and should be diluted before applying them to the skin. Mix a few drops of essential oil with a carrier oil, such as coconut oil or almond oil, to create a massage blend.

3. Add the Essential Oils to the Massage Blend: Once you've created your massage blend, apply it to your hands and massage it into the feet before beginning the reflexology treatment. The soothing scent of the essential oils will help relax the mind and body.

4. Use an Aromatherapy Diffuser: Another way to incorporate aromatherapy into your foot reflexology practice is to use an aromatherapy diffuser. Simply add a few drops of essential oil to the diffuser and let it fill the room with a relaxing aroma during the treatment.

5. Combine Reflexology with Aromatherapy: As you perform the reflexology treatment, take deep breaths to inhale the aroma of the essential oils. This can help enhance the relaxation benefits of the treatment and promote a sense of well-being.

6. Offer Aromatherapy as an Add-On: Consider offering aromatherapy as an add-on service to your foot reflexology practice. You can create customized blends for your clients based on their individual needs and preferences.

7. Educate Your Clients: Educate your clients about the benefits of aromatherapy and how it can enhance their foot reflexology experience. Provide them with information about the different essential oils and their properties.

By incorporating essential oils and aromatherapy into your foot reflexology practice, you can create a more relaxing and therapeutic experience for your clients and enhance the overall effectiveness of the treatment.

CHAPTER 6

Reflexology for Specific Conditions

Foot reflexology can be beneficial for a variety of health conditions.

Here are some ways in which reflexology can be used to support specific health issues:

1. Stress and Anxiety: Reflexology can help reduce stress and anxiety by promoting relaxation and reducing tension in the body. The calming effects of reflexology can help improve mood and promote a sense of well-being.

2. Pain Management: Reflexology can be used to help manage pain, including chronic pain conditions such as arthritis, back pain, and migraines. By stimulating the reflex points on the feet, reflexology can help reduce pain and promote healing.

3. Digestive Issues: Reflexology can help improve digestion and relieve symptoms of digestive disorders such as indigestion, bloating, and constipation. By stimulating the reflex points related to the digestive organs, reflexology can help promote better digestion and nutrient absorption.

4. Sleep Disorders: Reflexology can help improve sleep quality and reduce insomnia. By promoting relaxation and reducing stress, reflexology can help regulate sleep patterns and promote a more restful night's sleep.

5. Hormonal Imbalances: Reflexology can help balance hormones and relieve symptoms of hormonal imbalances such as PMS, menopause, and thyroid disorders. By stimulating the endocrine reflex points, reflexology can help regulate hormone levels and promote overall hormonal health.

6. Immune System Support: Reflexology can help strengthen the immune system and reduce the risk of infections and illnesses. By stimulating the reflex points related to the immune system, reflexology can help enhance immune function and promote overall health.

7. Pregnancy and Childbirth: Reflexology can be used during pregnancy to help reduce pregnancy-related symptoms such as nausea, back pain, and swelling. It can also be used to help induce labor and support the mother during childbirth.

8. Postoperative Care: Reflexology can help speed up the healing process and reduce pain and discomfort after surgery. By stimulating the reflex points related to the surgical area, reflexology can help promote healing and reduce inflammation.

It's important to note that while reflexology can be beneficial for many health conditions, it is not a substitute for medical treatment. It should be used as a complementary therapy to support overall health and well-being. Always consult with a qualified reflexologist or healthcare provider before beginning any new treatment regimen.

Using Reflexology for Pain Relief

Reflexology can be an effective tool for pain relief by targeting specific reflex points on the feet that correspond to different parts of the body.

Here's how reflexology can help alleviate pain:

1. **Stimulating Endorphin Release:** Reflexology stimulates the release of endorphins, which are the body's natural painkillers. Endorphins help reduce pain and promote a sense of well-being.

2. **Improving Circulation:** Reflexology helps improve blood circulation, which can reduce pain and inflammation in the body. Better circulation means that oxygen and nutrients can

reach the affected areas more efficiently, promoting healing.

3. Relaxing Muscles: Reflexology helps relax tense muscles, which can alleviate pain and improve flexibility. By targeting specific reflex points, reflexology can help release tension and promote muscle relaxation.

4. Reducing Stress and Anxiety: Reflexology promotes relaxation and reduces stress and anxiety, which are common contributors to pain. By calming the nervous system, reflexology can help reduce the perception of pain.

5. Balancing Energy Flow: Reflexology is based on the principle that imbalances in the body's energy flow can contribute to pain and illness. By stimulating the reflex points, reflexology helps restore balance and promote overall well-being, which can help reduce pain.

6. Specific Techniques for Pain Relief: Reflexologists use specific techniques to target pain relief, such as thumb walking, rotational pressing, and finger walking. These techniques help stimulate the reflex points associated with pain relief and promote healing in the corresponding areas of the body.

7. Complementary Therapy: Reflexology can be used as a complementary therapy alongside other pain management techniques, such as medication, physical therapy, and acupuncture. It can help enhance the effectiveness of these treatments and provide additional pain relief.

Overall, reflexology can be a safe and effective way to manage pain and promote healing in the body. It's important to consult with a qualified reflexologist or healthcare provider to determine if reflexology is a suitable option for your specific pain condition.

Reflexology for Stress and Anxiety

Reflexology can be a beneficial therapy for reducing stress and anxiety levels. By targeting specific reflex points on the feet, reflexology can help relax the body, calm the mind, and promote a sense of well-being.

Here's how reflexology can help with stress and anxiety:

1. Relaxation Response: Reflexology stimulates the nervous system to trigger the body's relaxation response. This response helps reduce stress hormones such as cortisol and promotes feelings of calmness and relaxation.

2. Release of Endorphins: Reflexology stimulates the release of endorphins, which are natural painkillers and mood enhancers. Endorphins help reduce stress and anxiety and promote a sense of well-being.

3. Improved Sleep: Reflexology can help improve sleep quality, which is often disrupted by stress and anxiety. By promoting relaxation and reducing tension, reflexology can help you achieve a more restful night's sleep.

4. Balancing Energy Levels: Reflexology aims to balance the body's energy flow, which can become disrupted by stress and anxiety. By stimulating the reflex points, reflexology helps restore balance and promote overall well-being.

5. Reduced Muscle Tension: Reflexology helps relax tense muscles, which is a common physical symptom of stress and anxiety. By targeting specific reflex points, reflexology can help release tension and promote muscle relaxation.

6. Improved Mood: Reflexology can help improve mood and reduce feelings of depression and anxiety. By promoting relaxation and reducing stress, reflexology can help lift your spirits and improve your overall outlook on life.

7. Complementary Therapy: Reflexology can be used as a complementary therapy alongside other stress-reducing techniques, such as meditation, yoga, and massage. It can help enhance the effectiveness of these treatments and provide additional stress relief.

Overall, reflexology can be a safe and effective way to reduce stress and anxiety levels and promote relaxation and well-being. It's important to consult with a qualified reflexologist or healthcare provider to determine if reflexology is a suitable option for managing your stress and anxiety.

Reflexology for Digestive Issues

Reflexology can be a beneficial therapy for improving digestive health and alleviating symptoms of digestive issues. By stimulating specific reflex points on the feet, reflexology can help promote better digestion, reduce bloating, and relieve symptoms such as indigestion and constipation.

Here's how reflexology can help with digestive issues:

1. Stimulation of Digestive Organs: Reflexology targets reflex points on the feet that correspond to the digestive organs, including the stomach, intestines, and liver. By stimulating these reflex points, reflexology can help improve the function of these organs and promote better digestion.

2. Relief from Bloating: Reflexology can help reduce bloating by stimulating the reflex points associated with the digestive system. This stimulation can help improve the flow of gas and relieve discomfort caused by bloating.

3. Regulation of Bowel Movements: Reflexology can help regulate bowel movements and relieve constipation. By stimulating the reflex points associated with the colon and intestines, reflexology can help promote better bowel function and reduce constipation.

4. Reduction of Acid Reflux: Reflexology can help reduce symptoms of acid reflux by promoting relaxation and reducing stress. By targeting reflex points associated with the esophagus and stomach, reflexology can help reduce the production of stomach acid and alleviate symptoms of acid reflux.

5. Stress Reduction: Stress is a common trigger for digestive issues. Reflexology can help reduce stress and promote relaxation, which can in turn improve digestion and reduce symptoms of digestive issues.

6. Complementary Therapy: Reflexology can be used as a complementary therapy alongside other treatments for digestive issues, such as dietary changes and medication. It can help enhance the effectiveness of these treatments and provide additional relief from digestive symptoms.

Overall, reflexology can be a safe and effective way to improve digestive health and alleviate symptoms of digestive issues. It's important to consult with a qualified reflexologist or healthcare provider to determine if reflexology is a suitable option for managing your digestive issues.

Reflexology for Sleep Disorders

Reflexology can be a helpful complementary therapy for managing sleep disorders by promoting relaxation, reducing stress, and balancing energy levels. By stimulating specific reflex points on the feet, reflexology can help improve sleep quality and regulate sleep patterns.

Here's how reflexology can benefit those with sleep disorders:

1. Stress Reduction: Reflexology promotes relaxation and reduces stress, which are common contributors to sleep disorders. By calming the nervous system, reflexology can help prepare the body and mind for sleep.

2. Calming the Mind: Reflexology can help quiet the mind and reduce racing thoughts, making it easier to fall asleep and stay asleep throughout the night.

3. Relaxing Muscles: Reflexology helps relax tense muscles, which can contribute to a more restful sleep. By targeting specific reflex points, reflexology can help release tension and promote muscle relaxation.

4. Balancing Energy Levels: Reflexology aims to balance the body's energy flow, which can become disrupted by stress and sleep disorders. By stimulating the reflex points, reflexology helps restore balance and promote a sense of calmness and well-being.

5. Improving Circulation: Reflexology improves blood circulation, which can help promote relaxation and reduce restlessness during sleep.

6. Complementary Therapy: Reflexology can be used alongside other therapies for sleep disorders, such as cognitive behavioral therapy for insomnia (CBT-I) or sleep medications. It can enhance the effectiveness of these treatments and provide additional support for better sleep.

7. Regulating Sleep Patterns: Reflexology can help regulate sleep patterns and promote a more consistent sleep-wake cycle. By stimulating the reflex points associated with sleep regulation, reflexology can help improve overall sleep quality.

It's important to note that while reflexology can be a helpful tool for managing sleep disorders, it should not replace medical treatment.

Always consult with a qualified reflexologist or healthcare provider to determine if reflexology is a suitable option for managing your sleep disorder.

CHAPTER 7

Reflexology for Special Populations

Reflexology can be beneficial for a wide range of populations, including children, pregnant women, and the elderly.

Here's how reflexology can be adapted for these special populations:

1. Children: Reflexology can be gentle and soothing for children. It can help promote relaxation, improve sleep, and reduce anxiety. When working with children, reflexologists use a lighter touch and shorter sessions to accommodate their shorter attention spans.

2. Pregnant Women: Reflexology can be safe and beneficial for pregnant women, especially during the second and third trimesters. It can help relieve common pregnancy symptoms such as back pain, swollen feet, and nausea. Reflexologists avoid certain reflex points that are believed to stimulate uterine contractions and focus on points that promote relaxation and balance.

3. Elderly: Reflexology can be particularly beneficial for the elderly, as it can help improve circulation, reduce pain, and promote relaxation. Reflexologists may use a gentler touch and focus on points that address specific health issues common in older adults, such as arthritis and circulatory problems.

4. People with Disabilities: Reflexology can be adapted for people with disabilities to accommodate their specific needs. Reflexologists can work with individuals in a seated or lying position, depending on their mobility. They can also focus on reflex points that address specific health issues related to the disability.

5. Cancer Patients: Reflexology can be a gentle and supportive therapy for cancer patients. It can help reduce pain, nausea, and fatigue associated with cancer treatments. Reflexologists work closely with healthcare providers to ensure that the treatment is safe and appropriate for the individual's condition.

6. Terminal Illness: Reflexology can provide comfort and support for individuals with terminal illnesses. It can help promote relaxation, reduce pain, and improve overall well-being. Reflexologists work with compassion and sensitivity to provide gentle and soothing treatment.

7. Dementia and Alzheimer's Disease: Reflexology can be a calming and comforting therapy for individuals with dementia or Alzheimer's disease. It can help reduce anxiety, improve mood, and enhance quality of life. Reflexologists use a gentle touch and focus on points that promote relaxation and mental clarity.

Reflexology can be a safe and effective therapy for special populations when performed by a qualified reflexologist. It's important to consult with a healthcare provider before starting any new therapy, especially for vulnerable populations.

Reflexology for Pregnant Women

Reflexology can be a safe and effective therapy for pregnant women, especially during the second and third trimesters. It can help relieve common pregnancy symptoms and promote overall well-being.

Here's how reflexology can benefit pregnant women:

1. Relief from Pregnancy Symptoms: Reflexology can help relieve common pregnancy symptoms such as back pain, sciatica, swollen feet, and nausea. By targeting specific reflex points, reflexology can help alleviate these discomforts and promote a more comfortable pregnancy.

2. Stress Reduction: Reflexology promotes relaxation and reduces stress, which is important for both the mother and the baby. By calming the nervous system, reflexology can help reduce anxiety and promote a sense of well-being during pregnancy.

3. Preparation for Labor: Reflexology can help prepare the body for labor by promoting relaxation and balancing energy levels. By stimulating specific reflex points, reflexology can help support the body's natural birthing process.

4. Hormonal Balance: Reflexology can help balance hormones during pregnancy, which can help reduce mood swings and promote emotional well-being. By targeting the endocrine reflex points, reflexology can help regulate hormone levels and promote overall hormonal health.

5. Labor Induction: Reflexology can be used to help induce labor naturally if the pregnancy is overdue. By stimulating specific reflex points, reflexology can help stimulate contractions and encourage the onset of labor.

6. Postpartum Recovery: Reflexology can be beneficial for postpartum recovery by promoting relaxation, reducing stress, and balancing hormones. It can help the mother recover from labor and delivery more quickly and support her overall well-being during the postpartum period.

When performing reflexology on pregnant women, it's important to use a gentle touch and avoid certain reflex points that are believed to stimulate uterine contractions. It's also important to consult with a qualified reflexologist or healthcare provider before starting any new therapy during pregnancy. Reflexology can be a safe and effective way to support a healthy pregnancy and promote overall well-being for both the mother and the baby.

Reflexology for Children

Reflexology can be a gentle and effective therapy for children, providing a range of benefits from relaxation to improved sleep. **Here's how reflexology can be beneficial for children:**

1. Calming and Relaxing: Reflexology can help children relax and reduce anxiety. It can be particularly helpful for children who are experiencing stress or have difficulty relaxing.

2. Improved Sleep: Reflexology can help improve sleep patterns in children. By promoting relaxation and reducing tension, reflexology can help children fall asleep faster and enjoy a more restful sleep.

3. Boosted Immune System: Reflexology can help boost the immune system in children. By stimulating the reflex points related to the immune system, reflexology can help improve overall health and reduce the risk of illness.

4. Improved Digestion: Reflexology can help improve digestion in children. By stimulating the reflex points related to the digestive system, reflexology can help promote better digestion and reduce symptoms such as bloating and constipation.

5. Pain Relief: Reflexology can help relieve pain in children. It can be particularly beneficial for children with conditions such as headaches, growing pains, or muscular tension.

6. Enhanced Well-Being: Reflexology can help promote a sense of well-being in children. By balancing energy levels and promoting relaxation, reflexology can help children feel more balanced and content.

When performing reflexology on children, it's important to use a gentle touch and adapt the treatment to suit their individual needs.

Reflexology can be a safe and effective therapy for children when performed by a qualified reflexologist or healthcare provider.

Reflexology for the Elderly

Reflexology can be a beneficial therapy for the elderly, helping to improve circulation, reduce pain, and promote relaxation.

Here's how reflexology can benefit the elderly:

1. Improved Circulation: Reflexology can help improve circulation in the feet and legs, which is important for overall health and mobility. By stimulating specific reflex points, reflexology can help enhance blood flow and reduce the risk of circulation-related issues.

2. Pain Relief: Reflexology can help relieve pain in the feet, legs, and other areas of the body. By targeting reflex points associated with pain relief, reflexology can help reduce discomfort and improve quality of life.

3. Relaxation and Stress Relief: Reflexology promotes relaxation and reduces stress, which is important for overall well-being. By calming the nervous system, reflexology can help reduce anxiety and promote a sense of calmness and relaxation.

4. Improved Sleep: Reflexology can help improve sleep quality in the elderly. By promoting relaxation and reducing tension, reflexology can help seniors fall asleep faster and enjoy a more restful sleep.

5. Enhanced Mobility: Reflexology can help improve mobility in the elderly. By stimulating reflex points associated with the feet and legs, reflexology can help reduce stiffness and improve flexibility.

6. Complementary Therapy: Reflexology can be used as a complementary therapy alongside other treatments for age-related issues, such as arthritis and circulation problems. It can help enhance the effectiveness of these treatments and provide additional support for overall health and well-being.

When performing reflexology on the elderly, it's important to use a gentle touch and adapt the treatment to suit their individual needs. Reflexology can be a safe and effective therapy for the elderly when performed by a qualified reflexologist or healthcare provider.

Reflexology for Athletes

Reflexology can be a beneficial therapy for athletes, helping to improve performance, reduce the risk of injury, and promote recovery.

Here's how reflexology can benefit athletes:

1. Improved Circulation: Reflexology can help improve blood circulation, which is important for delivering oxygen and nutrients to the muscles. By stimulating specific reflex points, reflexology can help enhance circulation and promote muscle function.

2. Reduced Muscle Tension: Reflexology can help reduce muscle tension and stiffness, which are common issues for athletes. By targeting reflex points associated with muscle relaxation, reflexology can help improve flexibility and reduce the risk of injury.

3. Faster Recovery: Reflexology can help speed up the recovery process after intense workouts or competitions. By promoting relaxation and reducing inflammation, reflexology can help the body recover more quickly and reduce muscle soreness.

4. Pain Relief: Reflexology can help relieve pain in athletes, such as muscle pain, joint pain, and headaches. By targeting reflex points associated with pain relief, reflexology can help reduce discomfort and improve overall well-being.

5. Stress Reduction: Reflexology promotes relaxation and reduces stress, which is important for athletes who may experience high levels of stress during training and competition. By calming the nervous system, reflexology can help athletes perform better and recover more effectively.

6. Complementary Therapy: Reflexology can be used as a complementary therapy alongside other treatments for sports-related injuries and issues. It can help enhance the effectiveness of these treatments and provide additional support for athletes' overall health and well-being.

When performing reflexology on athletes, it's important to use a firm touch and focus on areas of the feet and hands that correspond to the muscles and joints used during their sport.

Reflexology can be a safe and effective therapy for athletes when performed by a qualified reflexologist or healthcare provider.

CHAPTER 8

Integrating Reflexology into Your Life

Integrating reflexology into your daily routine can have many benefits for your overall health and well-being.

Here are some ways you can incorporate reflexology into your life:

1. Self-Reflexology: Learn basic reflexology techniques and perform them on yourself regularly. Focus on areas of the feet and hands that correspond to areas of the body where you may be experiencing discomfort or tension.

2. Regular Treatments: Schedule regular reflexology treatments with a qualified reflexologist. This can help you maintain balance and promote overall health and well-being.

3. Incorporate into Your Routine: Find ways to incorporate reflexology into your daily routine. For example, you can perform reflexology while watching TV, reading a book, or before bedtime to promote relaxation.

4. Use Reflexology Tools: Invest in reflexology tools such as foot rollers or reflexology socks to help stimulate reflex points and promote relaxation.

5. Combine with Other Therapies: Combine reflexology with other complementary therapies such as aromatherapy, massage, or acupuncture for enhanced benefits.

6. Stay Informed: Stay informed about the latest research and developments in reflexology to make informed decisions about how to integrate it into your life.

7. Listen to Your Body: Pay attention to how your body responds to reflexology and adjust your routine accordingly. If you experience any discomfort or pain, stop the treatment and consult with a healthcare professional.

By integrating reflexology into your life, you can experience a range of benefits, including reduced stress, improved circulation, and enhanced overall well-being. It's important to consult with a qualified reflexologist or healthcare provider before starting any new treatment regimen.

Self-Reflexology Technique

Self-reflexology is a simple and effective way to promote relaxation and well-being.

Here's a basic self-reflexology technique that you can try at home:

1. Prepare: Sit in a comfortable chair and remove your shoes and socks. Have a small amount of lotion or oil nearby if you prefer to use it.

2. Relax: Take a few deep breaths to relax your body and mind.

3. Start with the Toes: Using your thumbs, gently massage the base of each toe in a circular motion. Then, squeeze each toe gently between your thumb and index finger.

4. Move to the Ball of the Foot: Use your thumbs to apply pressure to the ball of your foot in a circular motion. Focus on any areas that feel tight or tender.

5. Work the Arch: Use your thumbs to apply pressure along the arch of your foot, moving from the heel to the ball of the foot. Use a firm but gentle pressure.

6. Massage the Heel: Use your thumbs to massage the heel of your foot in a circular motion. This can help relax the muscles and relieve tension.

7. Finish with the Ankle: Use your thumbs to massage around the ankle in a circular motion. Pay attention to any areas that feel tight or sore.

8. Repeat on the Other Foot: Repeat the same steps on your other foot.

9. Relax and Enjoy: After completing the self-reflexology technique on both feet, take a few moments to relax and enjoy the feeling of relaxation in your feet.

Self-reflexology can be a simple yet effective way to promote relaxation and well-being. It can be done regularly as part of your self-care routine to help reduce stress, improve circulation, and enhance overall health and well-being.

Incorporating Reflexology into Your Daily Routine

Incorporating reflexology into your daily routine can be a wonderful way to promote relaxation, reduce stress, and improve overall well-being. **Here are some simple ways to incorporate reflexology into your daily life:**

1. Morning Routine: Start your day with a few minutes of self-reflexology. Focus on stimulating reflex points on your feet that correspond to areas you want to energize for the day ahead.

2. Midday Break: Take a short break during your day to perform some self-reflexology. This can help refresh your mind and body, especially if you've been sitting or standing for long periods.

3. Evening Relaxation: Wind down in the evening with a longer reflexology session. Use this time to relax and de-stress before bedtime, focusing on reflex points that promote relaxation and sleep.

4. Before Bed: Perform a calming reflexology routine before bed to help promote a restful night's sleep. Focus on reflex points that promote relaxation and balance.

5. Incorporate into Other Activities: Combine reflexology with other relaxing activities, such as reading or watching TV. This can enhance the relaxation effects of both activities.

6. Use Reflexology Tools: Invest in reflexology tools such as foot rollers or reflexology socks to help stimulate reflex points throughout the day, even when you're not actively performing reflexology.

7. Mindfulness Practice: Practice mindfulness while performing reflexology. Focus on your breath and the sensations in your feet, allowing yourself to fully relax and be present in the moment.

8. Listen to Your Body: Pay attention to how your body responds to reflexology and adjust your routine as needed. If you feel discomfort or pain, stop the reflexology and consult with a healthcare professional.

Incorporating reflexology into your daily routine can be a simple yet effective way to improve your overall well-being. Whether you have a few minutes or a longer period of time to dedicate to reflexology, you can experience the benefits of this relaxing and therapeutic practice.

CHAPTER 9

Finding a Qualified Reflexologist

Finding a qualified reflexologist is essential to ensure you receive safe and effective treatment. **Here are some tips for finding a qualified reflexologist:**

1. Ask for Recommendations: Start by asking your friends, family, or healthcare provider for recommendations. They may know of a qualified reflexologist they can refer you to.

2. Check Credentials: Look for a reflexologist who has completed a comprehensive training program from a reputable school or institution. They should also be certified by a professional organization, such as the American Reflexology Certification Board (ARCB) or the Reflexology Association of America (RAA).

3. Verify Experience: Inquire about the reflexologist's experience and how long they have been practicing. A seasoned reflexologist with years of experience is likely to provide more effective treatment.

4. Ask About Specializations: If you have specific health concerns or conditions, ask the reflexologist if they have experience or training in treating those issues.

5. Check Reviews: Look for online reviews or testimonials from previous clients. This can give you an idea of the reflexologist's reputation and the quality of their services.

6. Visit the Facility: If possible, visit the reflexologist's practice to see the facility and meet the reflexologist in person. This can help you feel more comfortable and confident in your choice.

7. Ask About Hygiene and Safety Practices: Ensure that the reflexologist follows proper hygiene and safety practices, such as washing hands before and after treatments and using clean equipment.

8. Trust Your Instincts: Finally, trust your instincts. If something doesn't feel right or you're not comfortable with the reflexologist, it's okay to look for another practitioner.

By taking the time to find a qualified reflexologist, you can ensure that you receive safe and effective treatment that meets your specific needs.

Case studies and success stories are powerful tools for showcasing the benefits of reflexology. **Here are a few examples:**

1. Pain Relief: A case study of a client with chronic back pain who underwent regular reflexology treatments. After a few sessions, the client reported a significant reduction in pain and improved mobility, allowing them to resume daily activities with ease.

2. Stress Reduction: A success story of a client who was experiencing high levels of stress and anxiety. After incorporating reflexology into their routine, the client reported feeling more relaxed, calmer, and better able to cope with stressors in their life.

3. Improved Sleep: A case study of a client with insomnia who received reflexology treatments. After a few sessions, the client reported improved sleep quality and a reduction in the time it took to fall asleep, leading to a more rested and refreshed feeling during the day.

4. Enhanced Well-Being: A success story of a client who was feeling generally unwell and fatigued. After regular reflexology treatments, the client reported feeling more energetic, healthier, and happier overall, with a renewed sense of well-being.

5. Improved Digestion: A case study of a client with digestive issues such as bloating and constipation. After receiving reflexology treatments focused on the digestive reflex points, the client reported improved digestion and relief from their symptoms.

These case studies and success stories demonstrate the diverse benefits of reflexology and highlight its potential to improve the quality of life for individuals dealing with a variety of health issues. They can be used to inspire others to try reflexology and experience its positive effects firsthand.

Real-life examples of reflexology's impact can be found in numerous testimonials and personal accounts.

Here are a few examples:

1. Pain Management: Many individuals have reported significant pain relief from conditions such as back pain, arthritis, and migraines after receiving reflexology treatments. For example, a person with chronic back pain may find that regular reflexology sessions help reduce their pain levels and improve their overall quality of life.

2. Stress Reduction: Reflexology is known for its ability to promote relaxation and reduce stress. People often report feeling calmer and more at ease after a reflexology session, which can have a positive impact on their mental and emotional well-being.

3. Improved Sleep: Individuals struggling with insomnia or other sleep disorders may find that reflexology helps improve their sleep quality. By promoting relaxation and reducing tension, reflexology can help individuals achieve a more restful night's sleep.

4. Enhanced Circulation: Reflexology is believed to improve circulation, which can have a range of benefits for overall health. People with poor circulation may find that reflexology helps improve blood flow to their extremities, reducing numbness and tingling.

5. Digestive Health: Reflexology is thought to support digestive health by stimulating reflex points related to the digestive system. Individuals with digestive issues such as bloating, constipation, or indigestion may find relief from these symptoms after receiving reflexology treatments.

These real-life examples highlight the potential benefits of reflexology for a variety of health issues. While individual experiences may vary, many people find reflexology to be a valuable and effective complementary therapy for promoting health and well-being.

Client Testimonial: "I had been struggling with back pain for years and had tried numerous treatments with little relief. After just a few sessions of reflexology, I noticed a significant improvement in my pain levels. I was able to move more freely and without discomfort. Reflexology has been a game-changer for me, and I highly recommend it to anyone dealing with chronic pain." - Sarah

Practitioner Testimonial: "As a reflexologist, I have witnessed firsthand the transformative power of reflexology in my clients' lives. One of my clients was experiencing high levels of stress and anxiety, impacting their daily life and well-being. After a series of reflexology treatments, they reported feeling more relaxed, calmer, and better able to cope with stressors. It's incredibly rewarding to see the positive impact reflexology can have on someone's mental and emotional health." - John

CHAPTER 10

The Future of Reflexology

The future of reflexology is promising, with growing interest in holistic and alternative therapies for health and wellness.

Here are some key trends and developments that may shape the future of reflexology:

1. Integration with Conventional Medicine: Reflexology is increasingly being recognized as a complementary therapy that can be integrated with conventional medical treatments. As more research is conducted on the efficacy of reflexology, we may see greater acceptance and integration of reflexology into mainstream healthcare practices.

2. Technological Advancements: Technology is likely to play a role in the future of reflexology, with the development of tools and devices that can enhance the effectiveness of reflexology treatments. For example, wearable devices that provide biofeedback during reflexology sessions could help practitioners tailor treatments to individual needs.

3. Personalized Treatments: The future of reflexology may involve more personalized treatments tailored to individual needs. Practitioners may use techniques such as reflex mapping to identify specific areas of the body that require attention and customize treatments accordingly.

4. Research and Education: As interest in reflexology grows, there is likely to be an increased focus on research and education in the field. This may lead to a better understanding of the mechanisms behind reflexology and how it can be used to improve health and well-being.

5. Integration into Wellness Programs: Reflexology may become a more prominent feature in wellness programs offered by spas, wellness centers, and healthcare facilities. As people become more aware of the benefits of reflexology, they may seek out these services as part of their regular wellness routine.

Overall, the future of reflexology looks bright, with increasing recognition of its benefits and a growing demand for holistic and natural approaches to health and wellness.

Current trends and developments in reflexology reflect a growing interest in holistic health and wellness practices.

Here are some key trends:

1. Integration with Other Modalities: Reflexologists are increasingly integrating their practice with other modalities such as aromatherapy, acupuncture, and massage therapy to enhance the overall therapeutic effect.

2. Focus on Mental Health: There is a growing recognition of the role of reflexology in promoting mental health and well-being. Reflexology is being used to reduce stress, anxiety, and depression, and to improve overall mood and mental clarity.

3. Use of Technology: Some reflexologists are incorporating technology into their practice, such as using reflexology mapping apps to enhance their treatments and provide more personalized care.

4. Specialized Reflexology: There is a trend towards specialized forms of reflexology, such as facial reflexology and vertical reflexology, which target specific areas of the body or use different techniques to achieve therapeutic effects.

5. Research and Evidence-based Practice: There is a growing body of research supporting the efficacy of reflexology, leading to an increased emphasis on evidence-based practice among reflexologists.

6. Online and Remote Sessions: With the rise of telehealth and online wellness services, some reflexologists are offering virtual sessions to clients, allowing them to receive treatments from the comfort of their own homes.

7. Focus on Prevention and Wellness: Reflexology is increasingly being used as a preventive measure to maintain health and wellness, rather than just as a treatment for existing conditions.

These trends reflect a growing recognition of the benefits of reflexology and a shift towards more holistic and integrative approaches to health and wellness.

Research and studies supporting reflexology have grown significantly in recent years, providing a stronger evidence base for its effectiveness.

Here are some key findings:

1. Pain Relief: Several studies have shown that reflexology can help reduce pain in conditions such as migraines, back pain, and arthritis. A study published in the Journal of Clinical Nursing found that reflexology reduced pain and improved quality of life in patients with chronic low back pain.

2. Stress Reduction: Research indicates that reflexology can help reduce stress and anxiety levels. A study published in Complementary Therapies in Clinical Practice found that reflexology reduced stress and anxiety in women undergoing breast cancer treatment.

3. Improved Sleep: Reflexology has been found to improve sleep quality in various populations. A study published in the Journal of Alternative and Complementary Medicine found that reflexology improved sleep quality in postmenopausal women.

4. Enhanced Well-being: Reflexology has been associated with improved overall well-being and quality of life. A study published in Complementary Therapies in Medicine found that reflexology improved quality of life in patients with multiple sclerosis.

5. Pregnancy and Childbirth: Reflexology has been studied for its effects on pregnancy and childbirth. A study published in Midwifery found that reflexology reduced pain during labor and improved labor outcomes.

6. Cancer Care: Reflexology has shown promise in alleviating symptoms and improving quality of life in cancer patients. A study published in the Oncology Nursing Forum found that reflexology reduced fatigue in breast cancer patients undergoing chemotherapy.

7. Cardiovascular Health: Some studies suggest that reflexology may have beneficial effects on cardiovascular health. A study published in the Journal of Cardiovascular Nursing found that reflexology reduced blood pressure and anxiety in patients with hypertension.

While more research is needed to fully understand the mechanisms of action and long-term effects of reflexology, these studies provide support for its use as a complementary therapy for a variety of health conditions.

CHAPTER 11

Research and Studies Supporting

Research and studies supporting reflexology have grown significantly in recent years, providing a stronger evidence base for its effectiveness.

Here are some key findings:

1. Pain Relief: Several studies have shown that reflexology can help reduce pain in conditions such as migraines, back pain, and arthritis. A study published in the Journal of Clinical Nursing found that reflexology reduced pain and improved quality of life in patients with chronic low back pain.

2. Stress Reduction: Research indicates that reflexology can help reduce stress and anxiety levels. A study published in Complementary Therapies in Clinical Practice found that reflexology reduced stress and anxiety in women undergoing breast cancer treatment.

3. Improved Sleep: Reflexology has been found to improve sleep quality in various populations. A study published in the Journal of Alternative and Complementary Medicine found that reflexology improved sleep quality in postmenopausal women.

4. Enhanced Well-being: Reflexology has been associated with improved overall well-being and quality of life. A study published in Complementary Therapies in Medicine found that reflexology improved quality of life in patients with multiple sclerosis.

5. Pregnancy and Childbirth: Reflexology has been studied for its effects on pregnancy and childbirth. A study published in Midwifery found that reflexology reduced pain during labor and improved labor outcomes.

6. Cancer Care: Reflexology has shown promise in alleviating symptoms and improving quality of life in cancer patients. A study published in the Oncology Nursing Forum found that reflexology reduced fatigue in breast cancer patients undergoing chemotherapy.

7. Cardiovascular Health: Some studies suggest that reflexology may have beneficial effects on cardiovascular health. A study published in the Journal of Cardiovascular Nursing found that reflexology reduced blood pressure and anxiety in patients with hypertension.

While more research is needed to fully understand the mechanisms of action and long-term effects of reflexology, these studies provide support for its use as a complementary therapy for a variety of health conditions.

Final Thoughts on Reflexology

Foot reflexology is a holistic therapy that has been practiced for centuries and continues to be valued for its ability to promote relaxation, reduce stress, and improve overall well-being. It is based on the principle that specific points on the feet correspond to different organs and systems in the body, and by stimulating these points, balance and harmony can be restored.

Research has shown that reflexology can be beneficial for a variety of conditions, including pain, stress, insomnia, and digestive issues. It is often used as a complementary therapy alongside conventional treatments to enhance their effectiveness and promote healing.

Whether you're looking to improve your health, relieve tension, or simply relax, foot reflexology can be a valuable tool in your wellness toolkit. By incorporating reflexology into your routine, you can experience the many benefits it has to offer and support your overall health and well-being.

If you're intrigued by the potential benefits of foot reflexology, I encourage you to further explore this ancient practice. Consider trying a reflexology session with a qualified practitioner to experience the benefits firsthand. You may find that reflexology offers a unique way to relax, relieve stress, and support your overall health and well-being.

Additionally, consider learning more about reflexology techniques that you can use at home for self-care. There are many resources available, including books, online courses, and videos, that can help you learn how to perform reflexology on yourself or loved ones.

By exploring foot reflexology further, you can discover a holistic approach to health and wellness that may have a positive impact on your life.

Glossary of Key Terms

1. Reflexology: A holistic therapy based on the principle that specific points on the feet, hands, or ears correspond to different organs and systems in the body, and by stimulating these points, balance and healing can be achieved.

2. Reflex Points: Specific areas on the feet, hands, or ears that correspond to different organs, glands, and parts of the body.

3. Holistic Therapy: An approach to healthcare that considers the whole person – body, mind, and spirit – in the quest for optimal health and wellness.

4. Complementary Therapy: A non-mainstream therapy used alongside conventional medical treatments to support health and well-being.

5. Aromatherapy: The therapeutic use of essential oils extracted from plants to promote physical, emotional, and spiritual well-being.

6. Acupuncture: A traditional Chinese medicine practice that involves inserting thin needles into specific points on the body to stimulate energy flow and promote healing.

7. Massage Therapy: The manipulation of soft tissues in the body to improve circulation, reduce muscle tension, and promote relaxation.

8. Wellness: A state of complete physical, mental, and social well-being, not merely the absence of disease or infirmity.

9. Holistic Health: A approach to health care that considers the whole person – body, mind, spirit, and emotions – in the quest for optimal health and wellness.

10. Stress Reduction: Techniques or therapies designed to help reduce the physical and emotional effects of stress on the body.

11. Pain Management: Techniques or therapies used to help reduce or alleviate pain, often without the use of medication.

12. Well-being: A state of being comfortable, healthy, or happy, often used to describe an overall sense of wellness.

13. Homeostasis: The body's ability to maintain a stable internal environment despite external changes.

14. Energy Flow: The movement of energy throughout the body, believed to be essential for health and well-being in many traditional healing practices.

15. Meridians: Channels in the body through which energy flows, according to traditional Chinese medicine.

CONCLUSION

As we reach the end of our journey through the world of foot reflexology, it's time to reflect on the transformative power of this ancient practice and the impact it can have on our lives. Throughout this book, together we have explored the history, principles, techniques, and benefits of foot reflexology, gaining a deeper understanding of how it can enhance our health and well-being.

A Journey of Self-Discovery: Foot reflexology is not just about healing the body, it's also about connecting with ourselves on a deeper level. As we massage our feet and stimulate the reflex zones, we become more aware of our bodies and the subtle signals they send us. This awareness can lead to greater self-care and a more profound sense of well-being.

Empowerment Through Knowledge: One of the most powerful aspects of foot reflexology is its accessibility. You don't need expensive equipment or years of training to practice foot reflexology, all you need is your hands and a willingness to learn. By empowering yourself with the knowledge and techniques in this book, you can take control of your health and well-being in a whole new way.

Continuing Your Journey: As you continue on your journey with foot reflexology, I encourage you to explore further, experiment with different techniques, and listen to your body's wisdom. Remember, healing is a journey, not a destination, and every step you take towards wellness is a step in the right direction.

I invite you to integrate foot reflexology into your daily routine, using it as a tool to support your health and well-being. Whether you practice foot reflexology on yourself, with a partner, or seek out a qualified reflexologist, know that you are taking an active role in your health and wellness.

I encourage you to get a copy of the "Foot Reflexology Compendium " for yourself and even a friend or family member today. Let this book be your guide as you embark on a journey towards greater health, balance, and vitality. May your feet be a source of healing and strength, guiding you towards a life filled with wellness and joy.

www.ingramcontent.com/pod-product-compliance
Lightning Source LLC
Chambersburg PA
CBHW071013250726
48653CB00005B/1599